TABLE OF CONTENTS

CHAPTER ONE
PREFACE

The purpose of this book is to provide a guide for all catering both at home and for organizations. Its specific objectives is to prevent any outbreak of food poisoning as a result of unhygienic conditions in the food preparation chain. A food handler can be defined as a person who is involved at one stage or the other starting from the time of food buying, storage, transport, preparation or serving up to the time of consumption (eating). *"Clean food"*. *"Of course my food is clean, I would never serve dirty or tainted food"*. These are popular words from the food handlers. But, do you know that food which looks good can contain millions of germs able to cause disease called food poisoning? These germs are very small organisms that cannot be seen unless with the aid of microscope but they are present everywhere. This guide attempts to explain the causes of food poisoning and the principle of prevention.

Food poisoning is a disease as old as man. Some 3,000 years ago "Moses" instructed the Israelites in many hygienic principles and told them to wash their hands before eating. In the early days of man on earth, foods were cooked and eaten hot because there were not preservation method. But today most house wives and other food handlers buy their food in bulk weekly or monthly. They are taking advantage of modern preservation methods such as the refrigerators. Food is often cooked in bulk ahead of needs but the need for the provision of suitable facilities to enable food to be stored is not often considered.

The errors in food hygiene of large scale cooking often affect so many people at a time. But family cases are often unrecorded. An awareness of these problem and the means to combat them by careful measure is required

CHAPTER TWO

CONDITIONS FOR BACTERIA GROWTH

Germs can grow very rapidly and the more they are, the more the role they lay in making food bad for the health of those who eat it. Germs need five conditions to live and grow.

2.1 Suitable Temperatures (between 5°c and 50°c): Since **bacteria** grow in many environments from artic oceans to hot springs, it is not surprising that the **optimum growth temperatures** vary. **Bacteria** from the human gut grow well at body **temperature** (37 C) but **bacteria** from plants may be killed at that **temperature**.The body temperature 37°c encourages growth of most bacteria. The temperature in the kitchen is also favorable to them.

2.2 Food: All bacteria require energy to live and grow. Energy sources such as sugars, starch, protein, fats and other compounds provide the nutrients

2.3 Time: Germs like any other living things, need time to grow. Given the best conditions for growth one single germ can by dividing and re-dividing, producing up to 70,000 million germs in twelve hours.

2.4 Moisture: Moist foods encourage the growth of germs. Dehydrated foods allow survival but not growth of germs. Most germs do not multiply and grow at temperatures below 4°c and above 63°c, cold (even deep freezing) does not kill all germs, it merely prevents their growth. They are not killed by heat until temperatures above 63 are reached and applied for at least 10 minutes. Even this will not destroy the poison (toxin) which may be produced by some germs. Some of these germs form spores, which are heat resistant.

2.5 *pH* -- pH is a measure of acid or alkali in a product. It is indicated on a scale from 0 to 14, with seven being neutral. If the pH value is below 7, the food is classified as acid; if it is above 7, the food is classified as alkaline. Most bacteria grow well at neutral pH, but many can reproduce in a pH range from 4.5 - 10.0.

Although each of the major factors listed above plays an important role, the interplay between the factors ultimately determines whether a microorganism will grow in a given food. Often, the results of such interplay are unpredictable, as poorly understood synergism or antagonism may occur. An advantage is taken of this interplay with regard to preventing the outgrowth of the bacteria.

CHAPTER THREE
FOOD POISONING GERMS

There are many food poisoning germs. They are popularly called bacteria. Even these bacteria are of many types e.g. salmonella, staphylococcus, clostridium spp., etc. they cause the disease (food poisoning) by living organizing and multiplying within the food or by the release of a substance called toxin. These toxins are heat resistant. The consumption of food infected with such germs or toxins is the cause of such disease. The disease present symptoms such as fever, head ache, abdominal pain, diarrhea, vomiting etc. it is important therefore to know how germs reach our food.

3.1 Sources of Food Poisoning

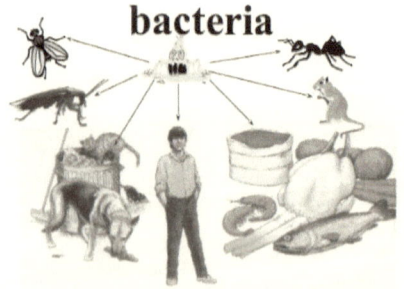

Sources of food poisoning bacteria

3.2 How Germs Reach Our Food

Germs can reach our food through

    a. Food handler

    b. Equipment and environment

    c. Water

    d. Pests

    e. Raw foods

3.3 Cycle of Infection and Contamination

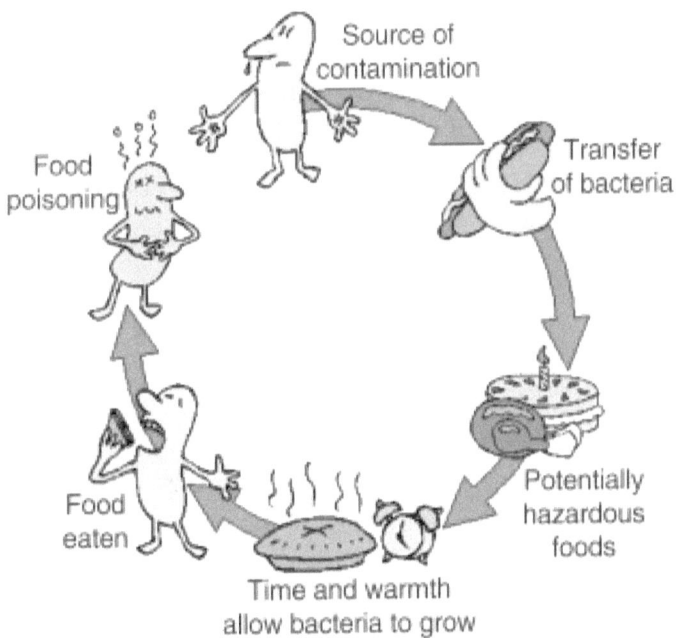

3.4 Food Handler

Germs are present in all parts of the human body. Careless handling during transport, storage, preparation and service may add germs to food. Hands can transfer food poisoning germs from raw to cooked food. Personal germs from the nose, mouth, skin, stool and hand can contaminate food. Wide spread of skin infections such as eczema not only render cleaning difficult but are connected with secondary germ infections

3.5 Equipment and Environment

Unclean kitchen surfaces and equipment can harbor germs and so contaminate foods; germs from raw foods e.g. meat can be passed to cooked foods. Dust and soil with dried excreta can contaminate food.
Disease such as typhoid fever, cholera, dysentery etc. are usually transmitted by water. Food can be also be contaminated with water.

3.6 Water:
Water contamination can occur by:
- By germs entering the water from the air
- By pests carrying germs into the water

- By coughing, sneezing, urinating and defecating directly or indirectly into the water

3.7 Pests:
Pests such as rats, cockroaches, flies can carry germs from different places such as toilet, dustbin etc. and bring them to our food

3.8 Raw Food:
Raw food such as meat, vegetables etc. carry a lot of germs. This can easily contaminate ready-to-eat-food once in contact with it

CHAPTER FOUR
CONTROL OF FOOD POISONING GERMS

It is good to control these germs so that they do not contaminate our food. Effective control should start from food buying, transport, storage, the environment where food is prepared (kitchen) and the food handlers themselves.

4.1 Food Buying

Since the relationship between germs, managed food stuffs are natural and constant, a careful thought should be given to the quality of the food we buy and the environment from where the food is bought.

- Buy only first class raw food with no physical evidence of spoilage such as odor, color change etc.

- Do not buy more than the quantity that your available preservation facilities can efficiently cope with

- Do not buy expired products

- Buy only hygienic food. To achieve this, a careful consideration should be given to the package materials, the environment and the person selling the food

4.2 Food Transportation

Food contamination can occur during transportation. Therefore, ensure that your food is transported under hygienic conditions

- Use vehicles with frozen storage facility for the transport of frozen foods

- Use vehicles with cold preservation facility for the transport of perishable food items for distance that will take up to 6 hours or more

- Wrap all ready-to-eat food such as meat pie, doughnut, etc. with clean foil paper before transportation

- Package canned foods properly to avoid denting during transportation. Denting brings the stored food with its container and could cause chemical food poisoning

- Do not transport food and chemical in the same vehicle. In fact, vehicle used for chemical transportation should not be used for food transportation

- Observe good hygienic practice during of loading

4.3 Food Storage

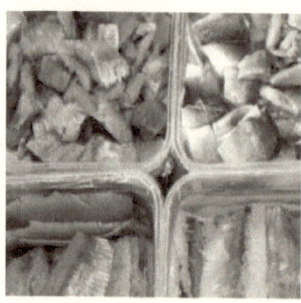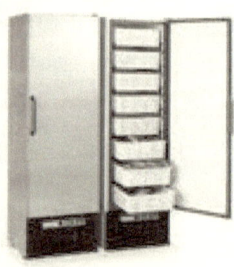

- Store food and food containers off the ground on shelves(at least 2.5cm above the ground)

- Raw vegetable should be stored separate from other perishable food, preferably in a separate store room

- Fresh fish must be kept separate, it taints other foods and leaking water will seriously contaminate other foodstuffs

- The principle of "first-in first out" should be strictly followed and checked. Where possible, food stuffs should be dated in order to ensure rotation

- For the preparation of meals, etc., no more perishable foodstuff must be taken from the cold storage than the amount which can be handled within the next hour. In hot temperatures the work time should be within a half-hour

- Prepared perishable products should be stored cold at temperatures between 2°c and 5°c or kept above 70°c until consumed

4.4 Storage of a Prepared Food

The method of storage after preparation may mean the difference between safe and unsafe food, the essential elements being time and temperature control. Food poisoning is seldom caused by contamination of food alone but such contamination plus the multiplication of the organisms, and this depends on the length of time the food is exposed to a temperature suitable for their growth. While all cooked prepared foods may be absolutely clean, it may not be possible, except at the time of heating, to guarantee their sterility. Because such Absolute sterility may be impossible, and because the subsequent safety or otherwise of that food will largely depend on the temperature at which it is stored, it is imperative to ensure that the period of storage between preparation and consumption is as short as possible, and that such storage will be at a temperature which will inhibit the multiplication of bacteria. It is therefore essential that:

a. All cooked foods must be cooled rapidly to a temperature of 5°c or below and remain stored at this temperature. All prepared dishes, whether to be served hot or cold, cold must be similarly stored. To achieve this, adequate facilities, both as regards space and refrigeration, must exist, and therefore no food preparation premises will be deemed suitable unless sufficient storage space with temperature of 5°c or below is available

b. Cold storage time should not exceed 24 hours (this limitation need not apply to frozen foods stored at lower temperatures). No perishable food should be served longer than 8 hours after leaving the cold store, unless an adequate method of refrigeration is provided.

c. No control of food storage possible without knowing the time of storage since preparation, and this is impossible without a system of time- stamping is introduced if safe storage is to be achieved

CHAPTER FIVE
REFRIGERATION OF FOOD

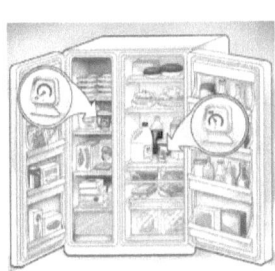 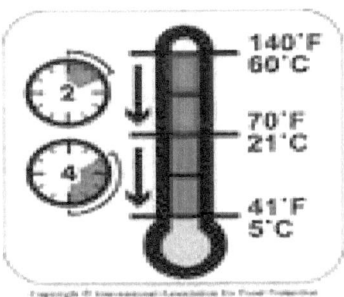

This is a common method of food preservation. The fridge temperature is between 2 and 8. As the temperature drops the growth of germs slow down. Perishable foods e.g. fresh tomatoes which are not for immediate consumption should be stored in the fridge. A common error responsible for the most cases of food borne disease, is to put a large quantity of warm food in the refrigerator. In an overburdened refrigerator, cooked foods cannot cool to the core as quickly as they must. When the center of food remains warm too long, germs grows quickly to disease producing levels

5.1 Correct Use of Refrigerators in Storage of Food

1. Do not overload- cold air must be allowed to circulate.

2. Store food below "load line" (chiller cabinet)

3. Store raw food below cooked food so that blood and juices cannot drip on to the cooked food

4. Use clean and recommended containers with lids rather than the original opened tins, for temporary storage of unused foods

5. Use tin foil, proof paper or polythene wrapping to prevent loss of flavor and transference of odors

6. Do not allow cooked food to cool for too long at room temperature before refrigeration or eating

5.2 Kitchen Control

-   Separate raw food from ready-to-eat food

-   Use separate equipment and surface for raw and ready-to-eat food

- Carry out thorough cleaning and disinfection of all surfaces, equipment and tools

- Apply cold storage of food to prevent multiplication of germs

- Institute personal hygiene

CHATER SIX
PERSONAL HYGIENE

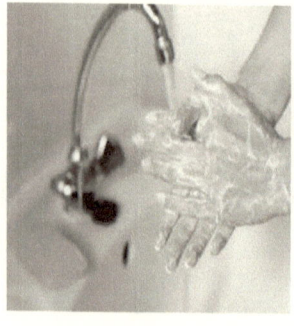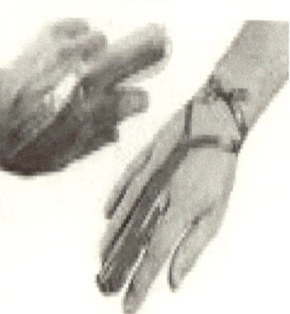

- Keep yourself clean

- Wash your hands thoroughly when you enter a food handling area

- Wash your hands thoroughly after using the toilet

- Wash your hands thoroughly after handling raw meat or dirty equipment

- Apply serious caution, if possible, do not handle food if you have any skin, nose, throat or bowel trouble, or any cuts or sores.

- Cover any cut with a clean water proof dressing

- Wear your protective or chef clothing properly and see that it is clean

- Make sure that your hair is completely covered

- Curb bad habit e.g. picking your nose, biting nails, licking fingers, dipping fingers in food.

- No smoking in any food room and was your hands after smoking in the rest room

- Do not eat in a room where food is prepared or stored

- Do not touch food more than is necessary

- Keep your finger nails short and clean

- When handling food do not wear jewelry which might harbor germs.

CHAPTER SEVEN
KITCHEN CLEANING METHOD

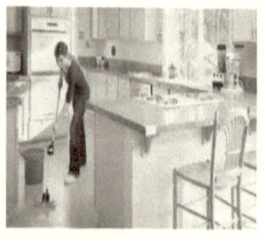 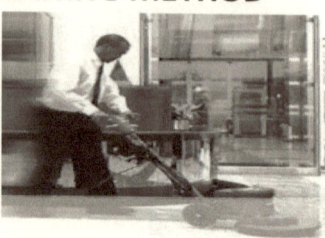

Dry sweeping of floors should be prohibited except to remove spilled items from small areas A careful cleaning of all parts of floors, non-food-contact equipment, wash basins etc., is to be preferred above casual cleaning procedures many times a day. The efficiency of dish washing machines depends on the correct temperatures of wash and rinse water and on the use of a correct concentration of proper detergent. Food container and other equipment should be cleaned with hot water at a minimum temperature of 82°C or with an appropriate disinfectant

7.1 Waste Disposal inside Kitchen

Food scraps on floors and surfaces encourage bacteria growth and attract vermin. Waste can be collected:

1. In pedal- operated bins which can be emptied regularly and washed out

2. In paper or plastic bags on pedal-operated stands. Bags can be sealed and put into dustbins and incinerated later.

7.2 Waste Management outside Kitchen

Provide sufficient waste bins or paper sacks to prevent over- spilling. Bins with well-fitted lids should be placed in a shade on a stand 250 to 300mm (10 to 12 inches) high above a concrete area with drainage.

CHAPTER EIGHT

HACCP PRINCIPLES/GUIDELINES

HACCP is defined as Hazards Analysis and Critical Control Point. It is a system that identifies and monitors specific food borne hazards- biological, chemical or physical that can adversely affect the safety of food. It involves the inherent risks attributable to a process or a product and then determining the necessary steps that will control the identified risks. HACCP systems are designed to prevent the occurrence of potential food safety problems. It is a food protection tool- evolutionary

8.1 PRNCIPLES OF HACCP

There are 7 principles of HACCP. They include:

1. Hazards Analysis

2. Identifying the critical control points in food preparation

3. Establish critical limits for preventive measures

4. Establish procedures to monitor critical control points

5. Establish the corrective action to be taken when critical limit is exceeded

6. Establish effective record keeping systems that document the HACCP system.

7. Establish procedures to verify that the HACCP system is working

8.2 Hazards Analysis

The hazards analysis process accomplishes three purposes

- Identifying all significant hazards

- Providing a risk- based frame work for selecting likely hazards

- Using the identified hazards to develop preventive measures for a process or product to ensure or improve food safety

8.3 Identifying Critical Control Point in Food Preparation

- A critical control point is a point- step or procedure at which control can be applied to prevent, eliminate or reduce a food safety hazards to as low as Reasonably practicable (ALARP)

- Points that may be control point in food preparation include cooking, chilling, specific sanitation procedure, product formulation control, prevention of cross contamination, and certain aspect of food handler and environmental hygiene

- Note that different facilities preparing the same food can differ in the risk of hazards and the CCPs.

8.4 Establish Critical Limits for Preventive Measures

- A critical limit is a criterion that must be met for each preventive measure associated with a CCP.

- It is a boundary of safety for each CCP and may be set for preventive measures such as temperature, time, physical dimension, A_w, pH and available Cl_2

- A CCP will have one or more preventive measures that must be properly controlled to ensure prevention, elimination, or reduction of hazards to ALARP

It is the responsibility of the food establishment to use competent authorities to validate that the critical limits chosen will control the hazards.

8.5 Establish Procedure to Monitor CCPs

- Observations and measurements

- Continuous monitoring

- Monitoring of procedure

8.6 Establish the Corrective Action Taken When Critical Limit is exceeded

o Determine the disposition of any food that was produced when a deviation was occurring

o Correct the cause of the deviation and ensure that the CCP is under control

o Maintain record of corrective actions

8.7 Establish Effective Record Keeping Systems that Document the HACCP System

▣ Written HACCP plan- requires the preparation and maintenance of a written HACCP plan by the food establishment detailing the hazards of each product

■ Record keeping- requires the maintenance of record generated during the operation of the plan; ensure preventive monitoring

■ Contents of the plan and records; approved HACCP plan and associated records must be on file at the food establishment

8.8 Establishment Procedures to Verify that the HACCP System Working

○ Carry out technical verification to ensure that Control Limits at CCPs are satisfactory

○ Verify that the facility's HACCP plan is working effectively

○ Carry out documented periodic revalidations independent of audits or other procedures to ensure accuracy of the HACCP plan

○ Bring regulatory agencies to ensure that the HACCP system is working satisfactorily.